EAT TO HEAL

Tase vikthor

Table of contents

Introduction

Open the door to delicious possibilities!

Forget bland meals and takeout nights. This cookbook is your key to unlocking a world of flavorful, nourishing dishes that fuel your body and tantalize your taste buds. Whether you're a seasoned chef or a kitchen newbie, these recipes are designed to inspire, empower, and make cooking a joy, not a chore.

Inside, you'll find:

Easy & Enticing: Mouthwatering recipes for every occasion, from quick weeknight dinners to show-stopping feasts, all packed with flavor and simple to follow.

More Than Just Meals: Explore chapters on mindful cooking, the link between food and well-being, and the power of sharing food with loved ones.

Fuel Your Life: Discover delicious dishes packed with essential nutrients, helping you feel energized, healthy, and happy.

Your Kitchen, Your Canvas: Experiment, personalize, and make these recipes your own. This is your guide to exploring the endless possibilities of food.

So grab your apron, gather your ingredients, and get ready to embark on a delicious adventure! Let's turn your kitchen into a haven of creativity, connection, and pure culinary joy.

Ready to get started? Flip the page and discover a world of flavor waiting to be explored!.

Chapter 1
Nourishing Foundations: Laying the Bricks for Your Recovery Feast

Imagine: a kitchen stocked with vibrant allies, a haven where meals become medicine, and flavors dance on your tongue, coaxing back your strength. That's what "Eat to Heal" is all about, and this chapter is your guide to building the perfect foundation for your culinary journey!

1.1 Building Your Recovery Pantry: Essential Staples & Smart Substitutions

Think of your pantry as your personal wellness war chest, stocked with allies to fuel your body and fight alongside you during treatment and recovery. Let's ditch the bland and boring, and fill it with vibrant ingredients that pack flavor and nourishment!

Essentials for Every Kitchen:

Grains: Quinoa, brown rice, farro, and whole-wheat bread provide lasting energy and fiber. Opt for gluten-free alternatives like millet or buckwheat if needed!

Proteins: Lean meats, fish, tofu, beans, and lentils offer essential building blocks for your body. Try skinless chicken, baked salmon, or lentil soup for variety.

Fruits & Veggies: Rainbow colored produce bursts with vitamins, minerals, and antioxidants. Stock up on frozen options for convenience, and don't forget leafy greens for extra power!

Healthy Fats: Olive oil, avocado, nuts, and seeds add healthy fats for energy and satiety. Sprinkle nuts on salads, use avocado in dips, or drizzle olive oil on roasted veggies.

Dairy & Substitutes: Go for plain yogurt, milk, and cheese, or explore plant-based alternatives like soy milk or almond cheese if dairy isn't your friend.

Smart Substitutions:

Gluten-Free: Swap pasta for lentil noodles, bread for gluten-free options, and thicken sauces with arrowroot powder instead of flour.

Dairy-Free: Use unsweetened plant-based milks in smoothies, coconut milk in curries, and top dishes with nutritional yeast instead of cheese.

Sugar-Conscious: Opt for naturally sweet fruits, use stevia as a sweetener, and choose unsweetened yogurt and nut butters.

Remember: This is just a starting point! Experiment, have fun, and personalize your pantry based on your taste, dietary needs, and preferences.

Next Up: Dive into the healing power of homemade broths and discover the superhero squad of cancer-fighting superfoods and spices in the next chapter!

1.2Broth is Beauty: Healing Power of Homemade Soups & Broths

Forget expensive store-bought cartons! Homemade broth is your secret weapon for delicious, nourishing meals that go way beyond just "comfort food." It's packed with flavor, hydration, and essential nutrients – a true gift to your body during recovery.

Why Broth is a Hero:

Hydration Powerhouse: Feeling drained? Broth is your answer! It's rich in electrolytes, like sodium and potassium, which help your body stay hydrated and keep things functioning smoothly.

Gut-Friendly Goodness: Broth is simmered for hours, extracting collagen and other nutrients that support your gut health. A happy gut means better digestion, immunity, and overall well-being.

Flavor Fiesta: Forget bland! Customize your broth with herbs, spices, and veggies for endless flavor combinations. Think ginger for a warming kick, turmeric for a golden glow, or your favorite herbs for a personalized touch.

Making Broth Magic:

Vegetable Broth: This is your versatile base. Roast your favorite veggies like carrots, onions, celery, and garlic, then simmer them in water for hours. Add herbs like thyme or bay leaves for extra flavor.

Chicken Broth (Cancer-Friendly!): Skip the store-bought options often loaded with sodium. Use lean chicken pieces, bones, and veggies, and simmer for hours. Remove the chicken and bones, and enjoy a light, flavorful broth.

Bone Broth: This powerhouse is packed with collagen, great for joint health and gut healing. Simmer bones from beef, chicken, or turkey with veggies and herbs for a rich, nourishing broth.

Pro-Tips:

Use a slow cooker for hands-off simmering.

Freeze leftover broth for quick meals later.

Add cooked broth to soups, stews, sauces, or even rice for extra flavor and nutrients.

Ready to unlock the healing power of homemade broth? Turn the page and discover delicious recipes to warm your body and soul!

1.3Fuel Your Body, Not the Disease: Cancer-Fighting Superfoods & Spices

Imagine your plate as a battlefield, and you're a warrior armed with delicious weapons! Instead of bland hospital fare, let's fill your arsenal with cancer-fighting foods and spices, packing powerful punches of flavor and nourishment.

Meet the Superfood Squad:

Rainbow Power: Stock up on colorful fruits and veggies. Berries boast antioxidants, broccoli fights free radicals, and leafy greens like spinach are packed with vitamins and minerals. Each vibrant bite supports your body's natural defenses.

Mushroom Mania: Don't underestimate these mighty fungi! Mushrooms like shiitake and maitake contain unique compounds that may help boost your immune system. Try them sauteed, grilled, or blended into soups for a savory boost.

Spice Up Your Life: Spices aren't just for flavor anymore! Turmeric curcumin boasts anti-inflammatory properties, while ginger can help ease nausea. Explore cumin, garlic, and black pepper - each with its own unique health benefits.

Spices: Your Secret Allies:

Turmeric: This golden wonder contains curcumin, a powerful compound with anti-inflammatory and antioxidant properties. Sprinkle it on veggies, add it to soups, or make a golden milk latte for a comforting treat.

Ginger: Feeling nauseous? Ginger to the rescue! This versatile spice soothes digestive woes and adds a zingy flavor to stir-fries, smoothies, and even tea.

Garlic: This potent allium vegetable packs a punch of flavor and immune-boosting power. Add it to roasted vegetables, sauces, or enjoy a simple garlic-infused broth.

Black Pepper: Don't underestimate this humble spice! Piperine in black pepper enhances the absorption of curcumin from turmeric, making them a dynamic duo in your kitchen.

Remember: This is just a taste of the incredible world of cancer-fighting foods and spices. Experiment, have fun, and discover what your body loves!

Next on the menu: Dive into simple substitutions for dietary needs and explore delicious recipes in the next chapter!.

Chapter 2

Comforting Classics, Reimagined: Where Nostalgia Meets Nutrition

Remember those childhood meals that warmed your soul? Chicken noodle soup on a rainy day, mac and cheese after a tough game, meatloaf smothered in gravy – pure comfort food magic. But what if we told you you can enjoy those same nostalgic flavors with a healthy twist? Buckle up, because this chapter is all about reimagining the classics, proving that delicious doesn't have to mean bland or unhealthy!

2.1 Chicken Noodle Nirvana: Lightened-Up Comfort Food for the Soul

Remember that steamy bowl of chicken noodle soup that always chased away the sniffles and soothed your soul? This recipe captures that comforting magic, but with a lighter, healthier twist!

Key Ingredients:

Lean Protein: Skinless, boneless chicken breasts or thighs, chopped.

Flavorful Broth: Low-sodium chicken broth, vegetable broth, or homemade broth for extra goodness.

Rainbow Veggies: Chopped carrots, celery, onions, and any other colorful favorites you like.

Whole-Wheat Noodles: For sustained energy and a satisfying bite.

Fresh Herbs: A sprinkle of thyme, parsley, or dill for a burst of flavor and aroma.

Simple Steps to Nirvana:

Simmer the Soul: In a large pot, combine broth, veggies, and your chosen herbs. Bring to a boil, then reduce heat and simmer for 15-20 minutes, or until vegetables are tender.

Shred the Hero: While the broth simmers, cook your chicken. You can poach it in the broth, bake it separately, or even use leftover rotisserie chicken for convenience. Shred the cooked chicken into bite-sized pieces.

Noodle Nirvana: Add whole-wheat noodles to the simmering broth and cook according to package instructions. Remember, al dente is your friend!

Protein Power: Once the noodles are cooked, stir in your shredded chicken and simmer for a few minutes to heat through.

Flavor Finale: Season with salt and pepper to taste, and don't forget that sprinkle of fresh herbs for an extra touch of magic!

Pro-Tips for Extra Comfort:

Add a dollop of plain Greek yogurt or cottage cheese for a creamy boost of protein.

Squeeze in some fresh lemon juice for a bright, tangy flavor.

Top your bowl with chopped fresh herbs, a sprinkle of whole-wheat croutons, or even a drizzle of olive oil for a satisfying finish.

Remember: This is just a starting point! Experiment with different vegetables, herbs, and spices to create your own personalized version of Chicken Noodle Nirvana. With a few simple swaps, you can enjoy this classic comfort food without sacrificing your health goals.

So grab your spoon, curl up with a warm bowl, and savor the taste of comfort, reimagined!

2.2Mac & Cheese Makeover: Creamy, Delicious, & Nutritious Twists

Who can resist the gooey pull and cheesy bliss of mac and cheese? But that heavy feeling afterwards? Not so cool. This recipe ditches the guilt without sacrificing the indulgence! Prepare to rediscover creamy, delicious mac and cheese packed with hidden veggies and protein – a win for your taste buds and your body.

The Key Players:

Veggies in Disguise: Roasted cauliflower, blended smooth, becomes your secret creamy base. Sneak in other veggies like zucchini or butternut squash for added vitamins and fiber.

Whole-Wheat Wonders: Ditch the refined noodles for whole-wheat versions. They provide sustained energy and a satisfying texture.

Cheesy Goodness (Reimagined): Reduced-fat cheese and low-fat milk keep things light, while nutritional yeast adds that cheesy flavor you crave.

Steps to Mac & Cheese Heaven:

Roast Your Veggie Hero: Preheat your oven and toss florets of cauliflower (or chosen veggie) with olive oil, spices, and a sprinkle of salt. Roast until tender and golden brown.

Blend it Creamy: Transfer the roasted veggies to a blender with some low-fat milk and nutritional yeast. Blend until smooth and luscious – your secret cheese sauce is born!

Noodle Time: Cook your whole-wheat pasta according to package instructions. Remember, al dente is key for a perfect bite.

Cheese Party (Light Version): In a large pot, combine your creamy veggie sauce, cooked pasta, shredded reduced-fat cheese, and a splash of milk. Stir gently until everything is coated in cheesy goodness.

Flavor Finale: Season with salt and pepper to taste, and if you're feeling fancy, sprinkle with some fresh herbs or a dash of paprika.

Pro-Tips for Extra Yum:

Add a scoop of ricotta cheese for an extra creamy texture without extra fat.

Stir in cooked, chopped broccoli or spinach for even more hidden veggies.

Top your creation with a sprinkle of whole-wheat breadcrumbs and bake for a few minutes for a cheesy, crispy crust.

Remember: This is your mac and cheese adventure! Experiment with different spices, add a pinch of hot sauce for a kick, or try different cheeses to find your perfect flavor combo. Enjoy the guilt-free satisfaction of creamy, delicious comfort food, made nutritious and delicious!

So grab your fork, gather your loved ones, and indulge in this healthier twist on a classic. Bon appétit!

2.3Meatloaf Magic: Lean, Flavorful, and Perfect for Picky Eaters

Forget the dense, greasy meatloaf of yesteryear! This recipe unleashes meatloaf magic, using leaner ingredients and sneaky tricks to create a juicy, flavorful loaf that's perfect for even the pickiest eaters.

The Lean and Mean Crew:

Protein Power: Lean ground turkey or chicken breast, chopped, is your protein base. Beef is okay, but choose lean cuts!

Moisture Magic: Grated zucchini or sweet potato adds moisture and hidden veggies without compromising taste.

Flavor Fiesta: Chopped onion, bell pepper, and mushrooms add savory depth and sneak in extra nutrients.

Fiber Fantastic: Whole-wheat breadcrumbs bind everything together and add a touch of fiber.

Spice Up Your Life: Herbs like thyme, oregano, and rosemary bring warmth and complexity to the flavor profile.

Abracadabra Meatloaf:

Prep the Veggies: Grate your zucchini or sweet potato and chop your onion, bell pepper, and mushrooms. Don't worry about them being perfectly uniform – variety is the spice of life!

Mix and Mingle: In a large bowl, combine your chosen protein, grated veggies, chopped vegetables, breadcrumbs, herbs, and an egg to bind everything together. Season generously with salt and pepper.

Shape It Up: Mold the mixture into a loaf shape on a baking sheet. You can use your hands (wet them first to avoid sticking) or a spatula.

Bake to Perfection: Preheat your oven to 375°F (190°C) and bake your meatloaf for about 45-50 minutes, or until cooked through. A meat thermometer inserted into the thickest part should read 165°F (74°C).

Flavor Finale: Let the meatloaf rest for a few minutes before slicing. You can brush it with a bit of ketchup or your favorite glaze for extra flavor, but it's delicious as is!

Pro-Tips for Extra Magic:

Add a handful of chopped nuts for extra crunch and protein.

Top your slices with a dollop of plain Greek yogurt or salsa for a cool and refreshing contrast.

Serve with roasted vegetables or a side salad for a complete and balanced meal.

Remember: This is your meatloaf masterpiece! Experiment with different spices, vegetables, and glazes to create your own unique flavor combinations. And don't be afraid to get creative with the presentation – even picky eaters will be drawn to a colorful and delicious-looking dish!

So grab your apron, gather your family, and prepare to be amazed by the magic of lean, flavorful, and irresistible meatloaf. Bon appétit!

P.S. Chapter 3 is all about satisfying your sweet tooth without derailing your health goals. Stay tuned for guilt-free treats that are as delicious as they are good for you!.

Chapter 3

Plant-Based Powerhouse Plates: Where Flavor Explodes and Vibrant Health Resides

Calling all plant-powered peeps and veggie-curious cooks! This chapter is your passport to a world of delicious, colorful, and nutritious meals that burst with flavor and goodness. Forget bland stereotypes – we're talking vibrant veggie bowls, protein-packed lentil creations, and one-pan wonders that make weeknight dinners a breeze. Buckle up, because we're about to show you how plant-based eating can be anything but boring!

3.1 Veggie Bowls of Bliss: Your Personal Flavor Fiesta in a Bowl

Forget boring salads and bland sides! Veggie bowls are your ticket to a symphony of flavor, color, and nutrients, all packed into one beautiful, customizable creation. Think of it as an artist's palette, where you get to choose the vibrant ingredients to paint your own masterpiece.

The Base Builders:

Grains for Energy: Quinoa, brown rice, farro, or even chopped romaine lettuce provide a hearty foundation for your bowl.

Greens for Goodness: Leafy greens like spinach, kale, or mixed greens add essential vitamins and minerals, plus a touch of freshness.

The Veggie Vibrancy:

Roasted Delights: Toss broccoli, carrots, sweet potatoes, or bell peppers with olive oil and spices, then roast until tender and caramelized for bursts of flavor.

Raw Power: Don't forget the raw veggies! Shredded carrots, cucumber slices, or cherry tomatoes add a refreshing crunch and extra vitamins.

The Protein Powerhouses:

Plant-Based Power: Cooked chickpeas, lentils, tempeh, tofu, or even a scoop of nut butter add protein to keep you feeling satisfied.

Eggs for Breakfast Bowls: Scrambled or poached eggs are a great way to add protein and richness to your morning bowl.

Creamy Companions:

Tahini Magic: Blend tahini with lemon juice, water, and a touch of garlic for a creamy, nutty sauce.

Hummus Heaven: Spread a dollop of hummus for a protein and fiber boost, or choose flavored varieties for a taste twist.

Avocado Bliss: Sliced avocado adds healthy fats and a creamy texture, plus a touch of vibrant green.

Flavor Finale:

Nutty Crunch: Sprinkle toasted nuts or seeds like almonds, sunflower seeds, or pumpkin seeds for added texture and healthy fats.

Herby Freshness: Chopped fresh herbs like cilantro, parsley, or dill add a burst of aroma and flavor.

Citrus Zing: A squeeze of fresh lemon or lime juice brightens up the entire bowl.

Remember: This is just a starting point! Get creative, experiment with different ingredients, and find what makes your taste buds sing. With a little planning and these tips, you can create veggie bowls that are:

Colorful and Eye-Catching: Feast your eyes on the vibrant colors of your creation.

Flavorful and Delicious: Each bite should be a burst of taste and texture.

Packed with Nutrients: Get your daily dose of vitamins, minerals, and fiber in one delicious bowl.

Customizable and Fun: Make it your own and discover endless possibilities!

So grab your favorite ingredients, unleash your creativity, and get ready to experience the bliss of veggie bowls!

Base Builders: Start with a sturdy foundation like quinoa, brown rice, or even chopped romaine lettuce.

Veggie Vibrancy: Roast colorful veggies like broccoli, carrots, and bell peppers for extra flavor. Don't forget leafy greens and fresh herbs for added vitamins and minerals.

Protein Powerhouses: Add cooked chickpeas, lentils, tempeh, or tofu for a satisfying protein punch.

Creamy Companions: Drizzle with tahini sauce, hummus, or a simple vinaigrette to tie everything together.

Flavor Finale: Don't forget the finishing touches! Sprinkle with toasted nuts, seeds, or a squeeze of fresh citrus for an extra burst of taste.

The beauty of veggie bowls? They're endlessly customizable! Swap ingredients based on what's in season, dietary needs, and personal preferences. Get creative, have fun, and discover your own bowl of bliss!

3.2Lentil Love: Your Hearty Passport to Protein-Packed Goodness

Move over, boring old soups! Lentils are here to transform your mealtimes with warm, flavorful creations that satisfy your soul and nourish your body. These tiny nutritional powerhouses are packed with protein, fiber, and essential nutrients, making them the perfect base for hearty soups and stews that are anything but bland.

Let's explore the delicious lentil landscape:

Spiced Lentil Soup: Imagine a warm hug in a bowl! This recipe combines lentils with warming spices like turmeric, cumin, and a touch of ginger, creating a cozy, flavorful haven perfect for chilly nights. Add chopped tomatoes, spinach, and a squeeze of lemon for extra depth and brightness.

Lentil Bolognese: Ditch the meat, not the flavor! This lentil-based "bolognese" is surprisingly meaty and satisfying. Simply simmer lentils with veggie crumbles, herbs, and your favorite tomato sauce. It's perfect for topping pasta, spaghetti squash, or even zucchini noodles for a lighter twist.

Curried Lentil Stew with Coconut Milk: Feeling adventurous? This creamy, flavorful stew takes you on a taste bud trip to the tropics. Coconut milk adds richness, while curry powder brings a warm, exotic spice. Throw in chickpeas, sweet potatoes, and your favorite veggies for a hearty and satisfying meal.

But lentil love doesn't stop there! These versatile legumes can be enjoyed in endless ways:

Soup it Up: Try lentil chili, lentil minestrone, or even a smoky lentil and sausage soup for a variety of flavor profiles.

Stew-pendous Creations: Get creative with lentil stews featuring Moroccan spices, Indian-inspired flavors, or even a hearty French lentil stew.

Salad Sensations: Toss cooked lentils with chopped veggies, herbs, and a light vinaigrette for a protein-packed salad that keeps you full.

Burger Bliss: Make lentil burgers for a healthier alternative to traditional beef patties. They're surprisingly satisfying and full of flavor.

Dip Delights: Blend cooked lentils with spices and herbs for a delicious and nutritious dip perfect for veggies or pita bread.

Remember: The key to lentil love is experimentation! Don't be afraid to try different spices, herbs, and ingredients to discover your own personal lentil masterpieces. With their affordability, ease of use, and nutritional power, lentils are sure to become a staple in your healthy and delicious cooking repertoire.

So grab your lentils, unleash your creativity, and get ready to experience the hearty satisfaction and endless possibilities of lentil love!

3.3One-Pan Wonders: Your Weeknight Savior with Veggie-Packed Flavor

Picture this: it's Wednesday night, the clock is ticking, and your energy is fading faster than the daylight. Enter the magic of one-pan wonders! These vegetarian sheet pan dinners are your ticket to delicious, stress-free meals that burst with flavor and clean up like a dream. Ditch the pots and pans, preheat your oven, and get ready to experience weeknight cooking bliss.

The Wonderful Basics:

Veggie Variety is Key: Choose a colorful mix of seasonal vegetables like broccoli, carrots, bell peppers, sweet potatoes, onions, or whatever strikes your fancy. Roasting brings out their natural sweetness and caramelizes them for extra flavor.

Protein Power: Don't forget the protein! Tofu cubes, tempeh crumbles, chickpeas, or even a sprinkle of nuts or seeds add a satisfying punch. Marinate your protein if you have time for extra flavor magic.

Flavorful Foundations: Don't just toss and roast! Toss your veggies and protein with olive oil, your favorite spices, herbs, or even a drizzle of balsamic vinegar for added depth.

Grains for Goodness: Serve your sheet pan creation over a bed of fluffy quinoa, brown rice, or even couscous for a complete and satisfying meal.

Recipe Round-Up for Busy Bees:

Rainbow Veggie Roast with Crispy Tofu: A classic for a reason! This dish lets the vibrant colors and flavors of roasted vegetables shine, while crispy tofu adds a delightful textural contrast.

Sheet Pan Fajitas: Sizzle and spice up your taste buds with this Mexican-inspired fiesta. Bell peppers, onions, and your choice of protein sizzle alongside tortillas for a quick and flavorful weeknight meal.

Lemon Garlic Baked Salmon with Roasted Asparagus: Feeling fancy on a budget? This elegant yet easy dish requires minimal prep and delivers maximum flavor.

Honey Mustard Glazed Chickpea Buddha Bowl: Toss chickpeas, broccoli, and sweet potatoes with a sweet and tangy honey mustard glaze, roast to perfection, and serve over a bed of quinoa for a satisfying and protein-packed bowl.

Remember: The beauty of one-pan wonders lies in their adaptability! Get creative, swap ingredients, and experiment with different spices and flavor combinations to find your own perfect sheet pan masterpieces.

Bonus Tip: Double the recipe and freeze half for another busy night! Just reheat in the oven and enjoy the convenience of a pre-made meal.

So ditch the stress, preheat your oven, and embrace the magic of one-pan wonders! These vegetarian delights are your key to healthy, delicious, and hassle-free weeknight dinners that will leave you feeling satisfied and ready to conquer your day.

Chapter 4

Sweet Treats that Don't Cheat: Where Indulgence Meets Nourishment

Forget the idea that healthy eating means sacrificing sweetness! This chapter is your passport to a world of delicious, guilt-free treats that satisfy your cravings without derailing your health goals. From breakfast delights that jumpstart your day to sweet endings that leave you feeling happy and satisfied, we've got you covered. So, grab your apron and get ready to experience the joy of treats that are both good for you and good for your taste buds!

4.1 Breakfast Bliss: Fuel Your Day with Delicious, Nutritious Treats!

Ditch the boring bowls of cereal and say hello to breakfast bliss! This chapter is bursting with recipes for muffins, pancakes, and smoothies that are not only mouthwatering but also packed with nutrients to kickstart your day in the best way possible.

Muffin Magic:

Rise and Shine Blueberry Muffins: Forget dry, store-bought muffins. These fluffy delights are bursting with juicy blueberries, whole-wheat flour for sustained energy, and a touch of sweetness from honey or maple syrup. Top them with chopped nuts or a drizzle of yogurt for an extra flavor boost.

Apple Cinnamon Spice Muffins: The warm aroma of cinnamon and the sweet-tartness of apples create a cozy and comforting muffin experience. Add a sprinkle of chopped walnuts for extra crunch and omega-3s.

Power-Up Protein Muffins: Looking for an extra energy boost? These muffins are packed with protein powder, Greek yogurt, and chia seeds for a satisfying and filling breakfast that keeps you going until lunchtime.

Pancake Paradise:

Whole-Wheat Banana Pancakes: Ditch the refined flour and embrace the fluffy goodness of whole-wheat pancakes. Ripe bananas add natural sweetness, while a touch of cinnamon brings warmth and flavor. Top with your favorite toppings like fresh fruit, nuts, or a drizzle of nut butter.

Oatmeal Raisin Pancakes: Packed with fiber and healthy fats, these pancakes are a delicious way to start your day. Oats add a satisfying chewiness, while raisins provide bursts of sweetness. Drizzle with maple syrup or honey for an extra treat.

Ricotta Spinach Pancakes: Looking for a savory twist? These protein-packed pancakes are made with ricotta cheese and spinach, creating a delicious and healthy alternative to traditional sweet pancakes. Top them with a dollop of Greek yogurt and a sprinkle of smoked paprika for a flavor explosion.

Smoothie Sensations:

Green Power Smoothie: Start your day with a vibrant green boost! Blend spinach, kale, banana, and your choice of milk for a vitamin-packed smoothie that's both refreshing and energizing. Add a scoop of protein powder for an extra kick.

Berrylicious Smoothie: Packed with antioxidants and immune-boosting power, this smoothie features a blend of berries, yogurt, and a touch of honey for sweetness. It's a delicious and healthy way to incorporate fruits into your diet.

Tropical Twist Smoothie: Transport yourself to paradise with this creamy and flavorful smoothie. Blend mango, pineapple, coconut milk, and a touch of ginger for a taste of the tropics. It's the perfect way to start a warm day.

Remember: These are just a few ideas to get you started! Experiment with different ingredients, flavors, and combinations to create your own breakfast bliss.

With a little creativity, you can enjoy delicious and nutritious breakfasts that will fuel your day and leave you feeling happy and satisfied.

So grab your apron, preheat your oven, and get ready to experience the joy of breakfast bliss!

4.2Guilt-Free Desserts: Sweet Endings That Don't Bite Back!

Craving something sweet after dinner but worried about the sugar crash and unwanted pounds? Fear not, dessert lovers! This chapter is your guide to indulging in delectable treats without the guilt or the dreaded sugar meltdown. We're talking satisfying sweetness that nourishes your body and leaves you feeling happy, not hangry. Buckle up for a guilt-free dessert adventure!

Baked Apple Bliss:

Cinnamon Swirl Apples: Remember those warm, gooey baked apples from your childhood? This recipe takes it up a notch with a sprinkle of cinnamon sugar, chopped nuts, and a drizzle of honey or maple syrup for a comforting and healthy treat. Plus, the fiber in apples keeps you feeling full and satisfied.

Apple Crisp with Oat Crumble: This classic dessert gets a healthy makeover with whole-wheat flour in the crumble topping. Feel free to experiment with different fruits like pears, peaches, or even berries for a variety of flavors.

Frozen Delights:

Frozen Yogurt Bark with Berries: Who needs ice cream when you have this? Layers of creamy Greek yogurt and fresh berries create a refreshing and delicious treat that's perfect for satisfying your sweet tooth without the heavy calories. Plus, you can customize it with your favorite fruit combinations!

Banana Nice Cream: This ingenious creation uses frozen bananas blended with a touch of cocoa powder or peanut butter for a creamy, dairy-free ice cream alternative. Top it with chopped nuts, granola, or even a drizzle of dark chocolate for extra indulgence.

Decadent Duos:

Dark Chocolate Avocado Mousse: Don't believe it? This creamy mousse uses avocados for richness and dark chocolate for that satisfying cocoa flavor, all naturally sweetened with a touch of honey. Top it with berries or a sprinkle of chia seeds for added texture and antioxidants.

Peanut Butter Chia Pudding: This protein-packed treat is made with chia seeds soaked in milk and blended with peanut butter for a creamy and delicious pudding. It's perfect for a quick and satisfying snack or dessert.

Remember: These are just a few examples to spark your creativity! Experiment with different ingredients, flavors, and textures to discover your own guilt-free dessert masterpieces. You might be surprised at how delicious healthy treats can be!

P.S. Looking for more inspiration? We've got you covered! Turn the page for delicious and healthy baking ideas that are perfect for satisfying your sweet tooth without compromising your health. Stay tuned for the sweet journey ahead!

4.3 Baking with Benefits: Cancer-Friendly Cookies for Sweet Satisfaction

For those navigating cancer treatment or recovery, even everyday indulgences like cookies can feel complicated. But fear not! This chapter proves that delicious cookies and mindful baking can go hand-in-hand, offering sweet treats specially formulated to be cancer-friendly. No compromise on flavor, just wholesome ingredients and minimized added sugar for guilt-free enjoyment.

Oatmeal Raisin with a Chia Seed Twist:

Remember those classic raisin cookies from childhood? This recipe gets a healthy upgrade with whole-wheat flour for sustained energy and fiber. We replace refined sugar with honey or maple syrup for sweetness, and add a sprinkle of chia seeds for extra omega-3s and crunch. Enjoy these soft and chewy cookies knowing you're nourishing your body with each bite.

Spiced Pumpkin Cookies: Warmth & Comfort All Around:

Fall vibes all year round! These cookies capture the essence of fall with warm spices like cinnamon and nutmeg, all while featuring the natural sweetness and vitamins of pumpkin puree. Whole-wheat flour adds a touch of fiber, and you can choose to use nut butter or seeds for added protein and healthy fats. Enjoy these cozy cookies with a cup of tea for a truly comforting treat.

Peanut Butter Banana Cookies: Protein Powerhouse:

Looking for a satisfying cookie that keeps you feeling full? These protein-packed cookies are made with whole-wheat flour, natural peanut butter, and mashed banana for a delicious and healthy combination. You can even add protein powder for an extra energy boost. These cookies are perfect for a post-workout snack or a satisfying afternoon treat.

Remember: These are just a starting point! Explore the endless possibilities of cancer-friendly baking by:

Swapping Refined Sugars: Experiment with natural sweeteners like honey, maple syrup, or even dates for a touch of sweetness.

Going Whole Wheat: Replace refined flour with whole-wheat flour for added fiber and nutrients.

Nuts & Seeds Power: Add chopped nuts or seeds for healthy fats, protein, and extra texture.

Spice Up Your Life: Experiment with different spices and herbs to create unique flavor profiles.

Portion Control: Enjoy these cookies in moderation as part of a balanced diet.

Baking with benefits doesn't mean sacrificing flavor or satisfaction. These cancer-friendly cookie recipes prove that you can indulge in delicious treats while being mindful of your health. So preheat your oven, grab your apron, and embark on a baking journey filled with flavor, care, and the joy of nourishing your body with every bite!.

Chapter 5
Cooking Through Treatment: Nourishing Your Body and Spirit

Navigating cancer treatment can be a whirlwind of emotions and physical challenges. But amidst it all, there's one thing that remains constant: the power of food to nourish your body and spirit. This chapter is your guide to cooking through treatment, offering delicious recipes that address specific side effects, adapt favorite dishes to accommodate sensitivities, and help you rebuild strength and vitality after treatment.

5.1 Managing Side Effects: Cooking to the Rescue!

Feeling drained by fatigue? Battling nausea that puts a damper on mealtimes? Taste buds acting up and making your favorite dishes unappealing? Don't worry, you're not alone! Cancer treatment can bring a whole host of side effects, but guess what? Food can be your secret weapon in managing them. Let's get cooking and show those side effects who's boss!

Fatigue Fighters:

Energy-Boosting Smoothies: Blend fruits, vegetables, and a scoop of protein powder for a quick and delicious pick-me-up. Think spinach, banana, and almond milk for a power-packed green smoothie, or berries, yogurt, and a touch of honey for a sweeter treat.

Hearty Soups & Stews: Warm, nourishing broths packed with protein and veggies are perfect for when fatigue leaves you with little appetite. Try lentil soup with chicken or turkey, or a creamy vegetable chowder with whole-wheat bread for dipping.

Nausea Navigators:

Ginger Power: This magical root is your friend! Add grated ginger to broths, stir-fries, or even sip on ginger tea for its calming properties.

Bland & Soothing: Stick to easily digestible foods like plain crackers, cooked rice, or mashed potatoes. Bland doesn't have to be boring! Add a squeeze of lemon or a sprinkle of herbs for a touch of flavor.

Small & Frequent Meals: Eating smaller portions more often can be easier on your stomach than large meals. Snack on bland fruits like applesauce or bananas throughout the day.

Taste Bud Twisters:

Mild & Mellow: Opt for milder flavors like cooked chicken or fish, steamed vegetables, and plain yogurt. Enhance them with herbs like parsley or dill for a subtle lift.

Texture Transformations: If strong textures are bothersome, try pureeing cooked vegetables or blending soups for a smoother consistency.

Experiment with Spices: Not all spices are created equal! Experiment with milder spices like turmeric, paprika, or cumin to add flavor without overwhelming your taste buds.

Remember: These are just starting points! Talk to your doctor or a registered dietitian for personalized advice on managing your specific side effects. And most importantly, listen to your body and choose foods that sound appealing and nourishing to you. Food should be a source of comfort and enjoyment, not stress, during this time.

So grab your apron, experiment with these tips, and discover how cooking can be your ally in managing treatment side effects. Feel empowered, nourished, and ready to tackle each day with a delicious bite!

5.2Chemo Cuisine: Comfort Food Favorites, Treatment-Friendly Twists!

Craving that warm, familiar lasagna that brings back happy memories? Or maybe a juicy burger is your go-to comfort food? Don't worry, just because you're undergoing treatment doesn't mean you have to give up these classics! This chapter is your guide to adapting your favorite comfort dishes to be chemo-friendly, ensuring you can still enjoy the flavors you love without compromising your health.

Lasagna Love, Lighter & Tastier:

Missing that cheesy, layered goodness? We've got you covered! Swap ground beef for lean ground turkey or chicken, use whole-wheat noodles for added fiber, and opt for reduced-fat ricotta cheese and mozzarella. Layer in plenty of veggies like spinach and zucchini for extra vitamins and moisture. You won't even miss the difference!

Burger Bliss, Lean & Mean:

Burgers don't have to be greasy indulgences! Choose lean ground turkey or chicken instead of beef, and bake or grill them for a healthier option. Pile on the toppings like lettuce, tomato, and onion for added flavor and nutrients. Swap the mayo for a dollop of hummus or guacamole for a creamy twist.

Mac & Cheese Makeover:

This classic comfort food can be easily adapted! Use whole-wheat pasta for fiber, and make a creamy sauce with low-fat milk, reduced-fat cheese, and a sprinkle of nutritional yeast for that cheesy goodness. Add roasted broccoli or cauliflower for a veggie boost.

Chicken Pot Pie, Cozy & Nutritious:

This hearty dish is perfect for a comforting meal. Opt for boneless, skinless chicken breasts, and use low-sodium broth for the base. Add plenty of colorful veggies like carrots, peas, and celery for vitamins and fiber. Top with a whole-wheat biscuit crust for a satisfying finish.

Remember: These are just a few ideas to get you started! Get creative and experiment with different ingredients and adaptations to suit your taste and treatment needs. Talk to your doctor or a registered dietitian for personalized advice on adapting your favorite dishes.

Most importantly, remember that food should be a source of comfort and enjoyment during this time. So grab your favorite recipes, make some healthy tweaks, and savor the deliciousness of familiar flavors with a treatment-friendly twist!

5.3 Post-Treatment Power-Up: Fueling Your Body for Renewed Strength & Vitality

Treatment is over, you've crossed the finish line, and now it's time to rebuild! This chapter is your guide to post-treatment power-up, packed with delicious recipes designed to help you regain strength, vitality, and celebrate your amazing journey. Think of it as fuel for your comeback!

Hearty Soups & Stews:

Lentil & Chicken Stew: This protein-packed wonder combines lean chicken with fiber-rich lentils, vegetables, and a flavorful broth. Perfect for chilly days or when you need a warm, nourishing hug in a bowl.

Minestrone Soup: This classic Italian soup is chock-full of veggies, beans, and pasta, providing a medley of vitamins, minerals, and fiber. Customize it with your favorite vegetables and lean protein sources like chicken or fish.

Protein-Rich Salads:

Grilled Chicken Caesar Salad: Skip the heavy dressing and opt for a simple lemon-herb vinaigrette. Add grilled chicken breast, cherry tomatoes, and crunchy romaine lettuce for a satisfying and refreshing meal.

Quinoa Salad with Black Beans & Corn: This colorful salad is bursting with protein from quinoa and black beans, while corn adds sweetness and fiber. Toss it with a light vinaigrette and enjoy a quick and energizing lunch.

Vibrant Stir-Fries:

Shrimp & Veggie Stir-Fry: Lean shrimp cooks quickly and provides essential protein, while a rainbow of stir-fried vegetables ensures you're getting a variety of vitamins and minerals. Serve over brown rice for a complete and flavorful meal.

Tofu & Broccoli Stir-Fry: This vegetarian option packs a protein punch with tofu and offers a good dose of vitamin C thanks to the broccoli. Add other veggies like bell peppers, carrots, and baby corn for added flavor and texture.

Superfood Boost:

Berry Smoothie Bowl: Blend your favorite berries with yogurt, protein powder, and a splash of milk for a creamy and delicious breakfast. Top with chia seeds, granola, and additional berries for an extra dose of antioxidants and fiber.

Salmon with Roasted Sweet Potatoes & Kale: Salmon is rich in omega-3 fatty acids, while sweet potatoes provide vitamin A and fiber. Roasting brings out their natural sweetness, and kale adds a dose of vitamins and minerals. A balanced and delicious post-treatment dinner!

Remember: These are just starting points! Experiment with different recipes, explore new ingredients, and discover what fuels your body and taste buds best. Focus on whole, unprocessed foods, lean protein sources, and plenty of fruits and vegetables for optimal recovery and sustained health.

Most importantly, celebrate your journey and honor your body with delicious, nourishing food! You've achieved something incredible, and now it's time to savor the taste of a healthy and vibrant future.

Chapter 6
Cooking for Two: Sharing the Journey, Plate by Plate

Cooking for two isn't just about whipping up meals; it's about creating experiences, igniting connections, and sharing the joy of food with those you love. This chapter is your culinary compass, guiding you through delicious adventures designed for two, whether it's a romantic rendezvous, a lively family gathering, or simply conquering your busy week with ease.

6.1 Date Night Dinners: Spark Joy & Connection with Every Bite!

Forget takeout and crowded restaurants! Create an unforgettable date night experience right at home with these romantic and delicious recipes designed to ignite the flames of love and connection. So, dim the lights, put on some tunes, and get ready to cook up some love on a plate!

Seared Scallops with Creamy Lemon Risotto: This elegant yet surprisingly easy dish is sure to impress. Imagine plump, perfectly seared scallops bathed in a zesty lemon sauce, nestled atop a bed of creamy, cheesy risotto – pure flavor magic! Here's how to make it happen:

Scallops: Pat them dry, season generously, and sear in hot oil until golden brown and just cooked through. Don't overcook, or they'll become rubbery!

Risotto: Toast arborio rice in butter, then gradually add warm broth, stirring constantly until creamy. Fold in Parmesan cheese, lemon zest, and a touch of cream for ultimate indulgence.

The Magic Touch: Plate the risotto, top with the seared scallops, drizzle with the lemon sauce, and garnish with fresh herbs for a restaurant-worthy presentation.

Herb-Crusted Rack of Lamb with Roasted Vegetables: This show-stopping centerpiece is perfect for a special occasion. Imagine a juicy rack of lamb crusted with a fragrant blend of herbs like rosemary, thyme, and garlic, roasted to perfection and served with a vibrant array of roasted vegetables – a feast for the eyes and the taste buds!

Lamb Prep: Combine your chosen herbs with breadcrumbs and Dijon mustard for a flavorful crust. Coat the lamb rack generously and roast until cooked through to your liking.

Vegetable Medley: Toss colorful vegetables like carrots, potatoes, and Brussels sprouts with olive oil and seasonings, then roast alongside the lamb for a delicious and healthy side.

Plating Perfection: Arrange the roasted vegetables on a platter, slice the lamb rack into individual chops, and drizzle with pan juices. Garnish with fresh herbs for a touch of color and aroma.

Chocolate Lava Cakes with Raspberry Sauce: End the night on a sweet note with these molten chocolate cakes that are guaranteed to steal hearts! Imagine warm, gooey centers bursting with rich chocolate, served with a tangy raspberry sauce – pure decadence!

Cake Magic: Whip up a simple chocolate cake batter and bake in individual ramekins. The key is to slightly underbake them so the centers remain molten.

Raspberry Bliss: Blend fresh or frozen raspberries with a touch of sugar and lemon juice for a vibrant and tart sauce.

Grand Finale: Plate the warm lava cakes, drizzle generously with the raspberry sauce, and dust with powdered sugar for an extra touch of sweetness. Prepare to be showered with compliments!

Remember: These are just starting points! Get creative, experiment with flavors and ingredients, and most importantly, have fun cooking together. After all, the most important ingredient in any date night recipe is love!

So grab your apron, put on your chef hats, and get ready to create a culinary love story that will leave you both wanting more!

6.2Family Feasts: Food, Fun, & Laughter Around the Table!

Gather your loved ones, crank up the laughter, and create memories that last a lifetime with these nourishing and crowd-pleasing recipes! Whether it's a birthday celebration, a casual weeknight dinner, or just a reason to get together, these dishes are guaranteed to bring joy and satisfaction to every plate.

One-Pan Roasted Chicken with Vegetables: The Easy Win:

Skip the stress and embrace simplicity with this fuss-free recipe. Imagine a juicy, golden-brown chicken nestled amongst colorful roasted veggies – all cooked in one pan for minimal cleanup and maximum flavor! Here's the magic:

Prep Party: Toss chicken pieces, potatoes, carrots, onions, and other veggies of choice with olive oil, herbs, and spices. Let everyone join in the fun!

One-Pan Wonder: Spread the mixture evenly on a baking sheet and let the oven do its magic. The chicken roasts to perfection, infusing the veggies with its delicious flavor.

Family Feast: Plate up the chicken and veggies, gather around the table, and enjoy a complete and satisfying meal with minimal effort!

Homemade Pizza Night: Get Creative, Get Messy, Get Delicious!

Turn pizza night into a family bonding experience! Imagine kids (and adults!) unleashing their inner pizzaiolos, creating customized masterpieces with their favorite toppings. Here's the recipe for fun:

Dough Power: Prepare a simple pizza dough recipe together. Let everyone knead, stretch, and get a little messy (it's all part of the fun!).

Topping Extravaganza: Set out a variety of toppings – classic pepperoni and mozzarella, adventurous options like roasted veggies and goat cheese, and everything in between!

Pizza Party Time: Let everyone build their own pizzas, bake them to golden perfection, and enjoy a meal that's as unique and delicious as your family!

Slow Cooker Pulled Pork Tacos: The Crowd-Pleasing Hero:

This recipe is perfect for those laid-back family dinners where everyone wants something satisfying and delicious. Imagine tender, flavorful pulled pork nestled in warm tortillas, topped with your favorite taco fixings – a guaranteed hit for all ages!

Slow Cooker Magic: Toss pork shoulder with your favorite BBQ sauce and spices, toss it in the slow cooker, and let it simmer all day. The pork will become melt-in-your-mouth delicious while you barely lift a finger!

Shredding & Serving: Shred the cooked pork with two forks, pile it high on warm tortillas, and let everyone customize their tacos with salsa, cheese, sour cream, and their favorite toppings.

Taco Tuesday Just Got Better: Enjoy a relaxed, fun-filled meal with minimal cleanup, leaving more time for laughter and family time!

Remember: These are just stepping stones on your family feast adventure! Explore new recipes, get creative with flavors and presentations, and most importantly, have fun cooking and eating together. Food is more than just sustenance; it's a way to connect, create memories, and celebrate the love that binds your family together.

So grab your aprons, turn up the music, and get ready to fill your kitchen with the aroma of delicious food, the sound of laughter, and the warmth of family!

P.S. Looking for more inspiration? Turn the page for tips on themed potlucks, picnic adventures, and engaging cooking activities that will turn your kitchen into a family fun zone! The culinary journey continues...

6.3Freezer-Friendly Favorites: Conquer Busy Days with Delicious Ease!

Life throws curveballs, and busy schedules can leave healthy eating by the wayside. But fear not, fellow time-crunched warriors! This chapter offers freezer-friendly recipes that are your secret weapons for conquering even the most hectic days. Imagine pulling out a delicious, homemade meal from the freezer, knowing you saved precious time and energy without sacrificing taste or quality. Let's dive in!

Make-Ahead Meatballs: The Versatile Hero:

These little flavor bombs are your freezer MVPs! Imagine whipping up a batch over the weekend, then tossing them into pasta, soups, stews, or even enjoying them on their own with a dipping sauce. Versatility is their middle name! Here's how to make them freezer-friendly:

Meatball Magic: Combine ground meat (beef, turkey, chicken, or a mix) with your favorite spices, herbs, and breadcrumbs. Form into bite-sized balls and bake until cooked through.

Freeze & Conquer: Let the meatballs cool completely, then flash freeze them on a baking sheet before transferring to freezer bags. This prevents them from sticking together.

Reheating Rhapsody: When needed, thaw meatballs in the fridge or microwave. Toss them into your favorite dishes for a quick and protein-packed boost.

Chicken Pot Pie Soup: Comfort in Every Bite:

This classic comfort food gets a freezer-friendly makeover! Imagine enjoying a warm, hearty bowl of creamy chicken pot pie soup, even on the busiest weeknight. Here's the recipe for freezer bliss:

Souptacular Creation: Simmer chicken, vegetables, and your favorite seasonings in a flavorful broth. Let it cool slightly, then portion it out into freezer-safe containers.

Freeze & Savor: Label and freeze your soup portions. When ready, thaw overnight in the fridge or heat directly in a saucepan.

Puff Pastry Perfection: For an extra special touch, preheat your oven and top the reheated soup with individual puff pastry squares before baking until golden brown. Comfort never tasted so good!

Breakfast Burrito Bowls: Fuel Your Mornings, On-the-Go:

Start your day with a nutritious and portable breakfast that tastes amazing! Imagine prepping these burrito bowls in advance, grabbing one from the freezer in the morning, and enjoying a delicious and satisfying meal without the rush. Here's the recipe for freezer-friendly mornings:

Scrambled Magic: Scramble eggs with your favorite breakfast fillings like sausage, peppers, onions, and cheese. Let them cool completely.

Bowl & Freeze: Divide the scrambled egg mixture into individual bowls, cover tightly, and freeze.

Morning Magic: Thaw a bowl overnight in the fridge or microwave in the morning. Serve over brown rice or quinoa, top with salsa and avocado, and fuel your day with freezer-friendly goodness!

Remember: These are just a few ideas to get you started! Explore different freezer-friendly recipes, experiment with ingredients, and most importantly, have fun creating meals that fit your busy lifestyle. With a little planning and these handy tips, you can conquer even the most hectic days with delicious, homemade food that nourishes your body and soul.

So grab your ingredients, get creative, and stock your freezer with delicious possibilities! The journey to conquering busy days, one delicious bite at a time, begins now!

P.S. Looking for more inspiration? Turn the page for tips on organizing your freezer, batch-cooking strategies, and even freezer-friendly dessert options! The possibilities are endless!.

Chapter 7
Beyond the Plate: Wellness in Every Bite

We've explored delicious recipes and filled your kitchen with mouthwatering aromas. But remember, food is more than just fuel; it's a powerful tool for nurturing your well-being in mind, body, and spirit. This chapter takes you beyond the plate, exploring how mindful cooking, understanding the link between food and health, and connecting with others through food can unlock a whole new level of wellness.

7.1Mindfulness in the Kitchen: Cooking as Self-Care

Remember that stressful feeling of rushing through dinner prep, chopping veggies on autopilot while your mind races between work emails and the grocery list? Yeah, we've all been there. But what if cooking could be different? What if it could be a form of self-care, a way to de-stress, connect with the present moment, and nourish your body and mind just as much as your plate?

Mindful cooking isn't about some fancy meditation session in your kitchen. It's about simple practices that bring awareness and intention to the act of preparing food. Think of it like a mini-vacation from the daily grind, a chance to reconnect with yourself and appreciate the present moment.

Here's how to turn your kitchen into a haven of mindfulness:

Breathe & Be Present: Before you even grab a knife, take a few deep breaths. Close your eyes, feel your feet grounded on the floor, and simply be present in the moment. Let go of distractions like your phone or TV, and focus on the task at hand.

Chop with Intention: Turn each action into a mindful practice. Feel the cool weight of the vegetables in your hands, listen to the rhythmic sound of the knife hitting the cutting board, and appreciate the transformation of ingredients into a nourishing meal. Notice the colors, textures, and smells – engage all your senses!

Savor Every Bite: Slow down! We often eat on autopilot, barely tasting our food. When you cook mindfully, the journey continues on your plate. Take small bites, chew slowly, and really notice the flavors and textures. Appreciate the effort you put into creating this meal, and nourish your body with gratitude.

Remember: This isn't about achieving some state of zen perfection. It's about bringing awareness and intention to your cooking experience. Even small mindful moments can make a big difference. Start with a few minutes of mindful breathing, focus on one task at a time, and gradually incorporate more practices as you feel comfortable.

The benefits? Reduced stress, improved focus, greater appreciation for food, and a deeper connection to the present moment. Not bad for simply being more mindful in the kitchen, right? So, next time you're cooking, take a deep breath, slow down, and enjoy the journey. Your body and mind will thank you!

Ready to explore more? Turn the page for tips on creating a calming kitchen environment, mindfulness exercises for busy cooks, and delicious recipes designed for mindful enjoyment. Bon appétit!

7.2 Food as Medicine: Nourishing Your Body from the Inside Out

Forget fad diets and magic potions! The real power to optimize your health lies right on your plate. Food choices significantly impact your physical and mental well-being, just like medicine impacts your body. This chapter dives into the exciting world of food as medicine, empowering you to make informed choices that fuel your body for a vibrant and healthy life.

Discover Nutrient Powerhouses:

Imagine your body as a high-performance engine. Just like a car needs the right fuel, your body needs specific nutrients to function optimally. This chapter introduces you to key nutrient powerhouses like:

Vitamins: Think A for vision, C for immunity, and D for bone health. Explore colorful fruits and vegetables, citrus fruits, and fatty fish for your vitamin fix.

Minerals: Calcium builds strong bones, iron carries oxygen, and potassium regulates blood pressure. Dairy products, leafy greens, and nuts are packed with these essential minerals.

Fiber: This gut-friendly champion aids digestion, regulates blood sugar, and keeps you feeling full. Load up on whole grains, fruits, and vegetables for a fiber fiesta!

Fuel Your Body for Life:

Ever felt sluggish after a heavy meal or energized after a light and healthy salad? That's the power of food choices in action! This chapter explores how different foods impact your:

Energy Levels: Sugary treats might give you a quick burst, but they crash hard. Opt for complex carbs like whole grains and lean protein for sustained energy throughout the day.

Mood: Feeling stressed or anxious? Certain foods can help! Omega-3 fatty acids found in fish and nuts have been linked to improved mood, while sugary treats can worsen anxiety.

Digestion: Feeling bloated or uncomfortable? Processed foods and sugary drinks can wreak havoc on your gut. Choose whole, unprocessed foods and fiber-rich options for a happy digestive system.

Balance is Key:

This isn't about strict restrictions and deprivation! It's about finding a sustainable and enjoyable approach to food. This chapter emphasizes:

Mindful Indulgence: Enjoying occasional treats is part of a balanced lifestyle. Savor those birthday cake bites or ice cream cones, but make them mindful choices, not daily habits.

Portion Control: It's not just what you eat, but how much. Learn about healthy portion sizes and listen to your body's hunger cues to avoid overeating.

Variety is the Spice of Life (and Health!): Explore different cuisines, fruits, and vegetables to ensure your body gets a wide range of nutrients and keeps your taste buds happy.

Remember: You're the chef of your own health! This chapter is just the starting point. Explore resources like cookbooks, websites, and even consult a registered dietitian for personalized guidance. With knowledge, mindful choices, and a dash of deliciousness, you can use food as your powerful ally for a healthy and vibrant life!.

Conclusion

The Recipe for a Life Well-Nourished:

As you reach the end of this culinary adventure, remember, this book is just the beginning. It's not just a collection of recipes; it's an invitation to explore, experiment, and discover the joy of cooking and eating with intention.

You've learned about delicious dishes to share with loved ones, quick fixes for busy days, and even mindful practices to turn cooking into self-care. But the most important ingredient you've gained is knowledge – knowledge about the power of food to nourish your body, connect you to others, and fuel your journey towards a healthier, happier you.

So, what's next?

Keep exploring: Don't be afraid to step outside your comfort zone and try new cuisines, ingredients, and cooking techniques. The world of food is vast and exciting!

Share the love: Cooking is meant to be shared. Gather your friends and family, host potlucks, or simply cook together and enjoy the laughter and connection that comes with sharing a meal.

Listen to your body: Pay attention to how different foods make you feel. What gives you energy? What leaves you sluggish? Experiment and find what works best for you.

Make it fun! Cooking shouldn't be a chore. Put on some music, dance around the kitchen, and embrace the joy of creating something delicious.

Remember, you are the author of your own culinary story. Use the recipes in this book as inspiration, but don't be afraid to write your own chapters. Experiment, have fun, and most importantly, never stop exploring the delicious possibilities that food has to offer!

Here are some final thoughts to leave you with:

Food is more than just fuel; it's an experience, a connection, and a celebration of life.

Cooking is a creative outlet, a stress reliever, and a way to express yourself.

Sharing food with others strengthens bonds and creates lasting memories.

Nourishing your body with delicious, wholesome food is an act of self-love.

So, put on your apron, grab your favorite ingredients, and get ready to create something amazing! The kitchen is your canvas, and the possibilities are endless.

Bon appétit, and happy cooking!.